EYE AND VISION RESEARCH DEVELOPMENTS

EYE DISEASES AND DISORDERS

WHAT YOU SHOULD KNOW

EYE AND VISION RESEARCH DEVELOPMENTS

Additional books in this series can be found on Nova's website under the Series tab.

Additional e-books in this series can be found on Nova's website under the e-book tab.

EYE AND VISION RESEARCH DEVELOPMENTS

EYE DISEASES AND DISORDERS
WHAT YOU SHOULD KNOW

RACHAEL GRAY
EDITOR

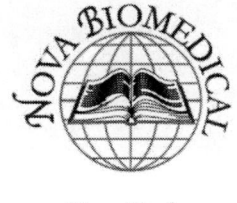

New York

Copyright © 2015 by Nova Science Publishers, Inc.

All rights reserved. No part of this book may be reproduced, stored in a retrieval system or transmitted in any form or by any means: electronic, electrostatic, magnetic, tape, mechanical photocopying, recording or otherwise without the written permission of the Publisher.

For permission to use material from this book please contact us:
nova.main@novapublishers.com

NOTICE TO THE READER

The Publisher has taken reasonable care in the preparation of this book, but makes no expressed or implied warranty of any kind and assumes no responsibility for any errors or omissions. No liability is assumed for incidental or consequential damages in connection with or arising out of information contained in this book. The Publisher shall not be liable for any special, consequential, or exemplary damages resulting, in whole or in part, from the readers' use of, or reliance upon, this material. Any parts of this book based on government reports are so indicated and copyright is claimed for those parts to the extent applicable to compilations of such works.

Independent verification should be sought for any data, advice or recommendations contained in this book. In addition, no responsibility is assumed by the publisher for any injury and/or damage to persons or property arising from any methods, products, instructions, ideas or otherwise contained in this publication.

This publication is designed to provide accurate and authoritative information with regard to the subject matter covered herein. It is sold with the clear understanding that the Publisher is not engaged in rendering legal or any other professional services. If legal or any other expert assistance is required, the services of a competent person should be sought. FROM A DECLARATION OF PARTICIPANTS JOINTLY ADOPTED BY A COMMITTEE OF THE AMERICAN BAR ASSOCIATION AND A COMMITTEE OF PUBLISHERS.

Additional color graphics may be available in the e-book version of this book.

Library of Congress Cataloging-in-Publication Data

ISBN: 978-1-63463-895-1

Published by Nova Science Publishers, Inc. † New York

Contents

Preface		**vii**
Chapter 1	Glaucoma: What You Should Know *National Eye Institute*	**1**
Chapter 2	Cataract: What You Should Know *National Eye Institute*	**17**
Chapter 3	Age-Related Macular Degeneration: What You Should Know *National Eye Institute*	**31**
Chapter 4	Diabetic Retinopathy: What You Should Know *National Eye Institute*	**47**
Index		**61**

Preface

Chapter 1 – This chapter is for people with glaucoma and their families and friends. It provides information about open-angle glaucoma, the most common form of glaucoma. This chapter answers questions about the cause and symptoms of the disease and discusses diagnosis and types of treatment.

Chapter 2 – This chapter is for people with cataract and their families and friends. It provides information about age-related cataract, the most common form of cataract. This chapter answers questions about the causes and symptoms of the disorder and discusses diagnosis and types of treatment.

Chapter 3 – This chapter is for people with age-related macular degeneration (AMD) and their families and friends. It provides information about AMD and answers questions about its causes and symptoms. Diagnosis and types of treatment are described.

Chapter 4 – This chapter is for people with diabetic retinopathy and their families and friends. It provides information about diabetic retinopathy and answers questions about the cause and symptoms of this progressive eye disease. Diagnosis and types of treatment are described.

In: Eye Diseases and Disorders
Editor: Rachael Gray

ISBN: 978-1-63463-895-1
© 2015 Nova Science Publishers, Inc.

Chapter 1

Glaucoma: What You Should Know[*]

National Eye Institute

What You Should Know About Glaucoma

This chapter is for people with glaucoma and their families and friends. It provides information about open-angle glaucoma, the most common form of glaucoma. This chapter answers questions about the causes and symptoms of this disease and discusses diagnosis and types of treatment.

What Is Glaucoma?

Glaucoma is a group of diseases that damage the eye's optic nerve and can result in vision loss and blindness. However, with early detection and treatment, you can often protect your eyes against serious vision loss.

---

[*] This is an edited, reformatted and augmented version of a document (revised November 2014) issued by the National Institutes of Health, National Eye Institute.

The Optic Nerve

The optic nerve is a bundle of more than 1 million nerve fibers. It connects the retina to the brain. (See diagram below.) The retina is the light-sensitive tissue at the back of the eye. A healthy optic nerve is necessary for good vision.

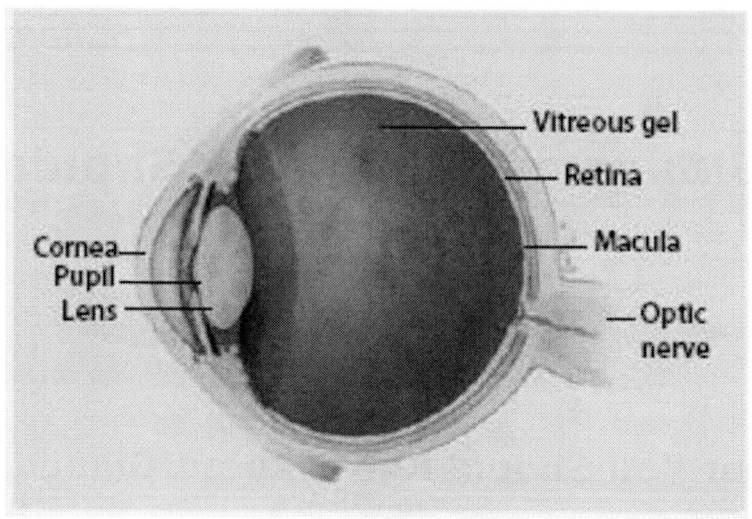

How Does the Optic Nerve Get Damaged by Open-Angle Glaucoma?

Several large studies have shown that eye pressure is a major risk factor for optic nerve damage. In the front of the eye is a space called the anterior chamber. A clear fluid flows continuously in and out of the chamber and nourishes nearby tissues. The fluid leaves the chamber at the open angle where the cornea and iris meet. (See diagram below.) When the fluid reaches the angle, it flows through a spongy meshwork, like a drain, and leaves the eye.

In open-angle glaucoma, even though the drainage angle is "open," the fluid passes too slowly through the meshwork drain. Since the fluid builds up, the pressure inside the eye rises to a level that may damage the optic nerve. When the optic nerve is damaged from increased pressure, open-angle glaucoma—and vision loss—may result. That's why controlling pressure inside the eye is important.

Another risk factor for optic nerve damage relates to blood pressure. Thus, it is important to also make sure that your blood pressure is at a proper level for your body by working with your medical doctor.

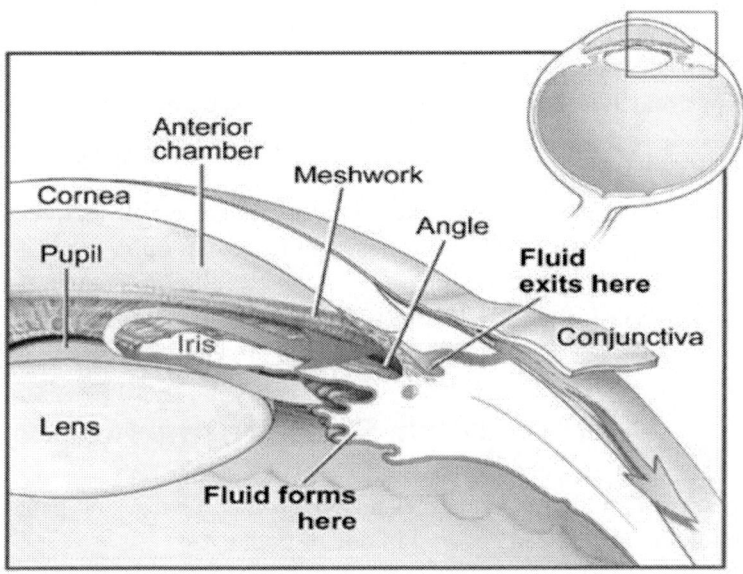

Can I Develop Glaucoma if I Have Increased Eye Pressure?

Not necessarily. Not every person with increased eye pressure will develop glaucoma. Some people can tolerate higher levels of eye pressure better than others. Also, a certain level of eye pressure may be high for one person but normal for another.

Whether you develop glaucoma depends on the level of pressure your optic nerve can tolerate without being damaged. This level is different for each person. That's why a comprehensive dilated eye exam is very important. It can help your eye care professional determine what level of eye pressure is normal for you.

Can I Develop Glaucoma without an Increase in My Eye Pressure?

Yes. Glaucoma can develop without increased eye pressure. This form of glaucoma is called low-tension or normal-tension glaucoma. It is a type of open-angle glaucoma.

Who Is at Risk for Open-Angle Glaucoma?

Anyone can develop glaucoma. Some people, listed below, are at higher risk than others:

- African Americans over age 40
- Everyone over age 60, especially Hispanics/Latinos
- People with a family history of glaucoma

A comprehensive dilated eye exam can reveal more risk factors, such as high eye pressure, thinness of the cornea, and abnormal optic nerve anatomy. In some people with certain combinations of these high-risk factors, medicines in the form of eyedrops reduce the risk of developing glaucoma by about half.

Glaucoma Symptoms

At first, open-angle glaucoma has no symptoms. It causes no pain. Vision stays normal. Glaucoma can develop in one or both eyes.

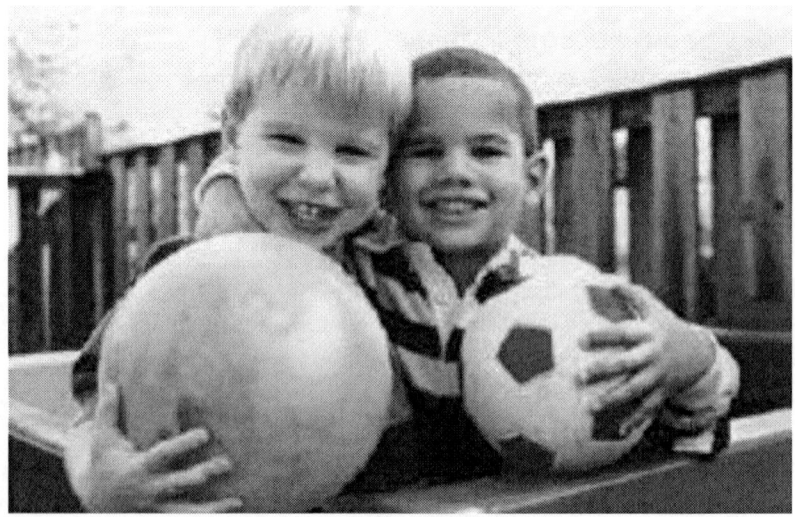

Normal vision

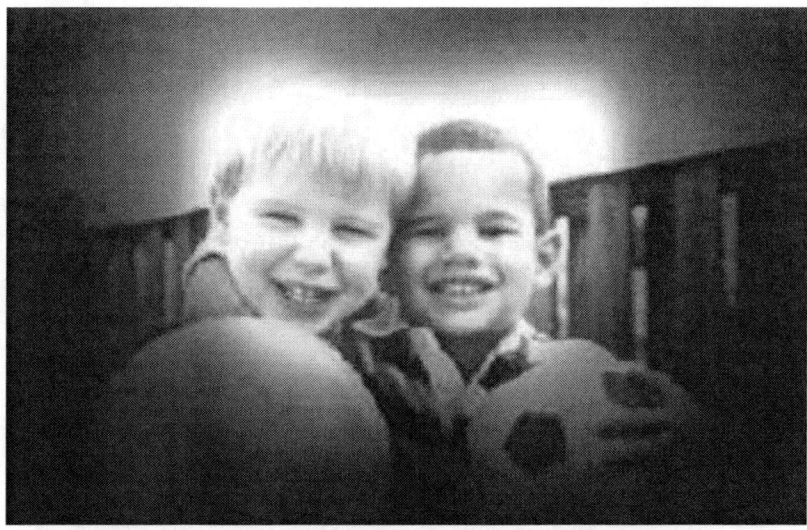

The same scene as viewed by a person with glaucoma

Without treatment, people with glaucoma will slowly lose their peripheral (side) vision. As glaucoma remains untreated, people may miss objects to the side and out of the corner of their eye. They seem to be looking through a tunnel. Over time, straight-ahead (central) vision may decrease until no vision remains.

How Is Glaucoma Detected?

Glaucoma is detected through a comprehensive dilated eye exam that includes the following:

Visual Acuity Test
This eye chart test measures how well you see at various distances.

Visual Field Test
This test measures your peripheral (side vision). It helps your eye care professional tell if you have lost peripheral vision, a sign of glaucoma.

Dilated Eye Exam

In this exam, drops are placed in your eyes to widen, or dilate, the pupils. Your eye care professional uses a special magnifying lens to examine your retina and optic nerve for signs of damage and other eye problems. After the exam, your close-up vision may remain blurred for several hours.

Tonometry is the measurement of pressure inside the eye by using an instrument (right) called a tonometer. Numbing drops may be applied to your eye for this test.

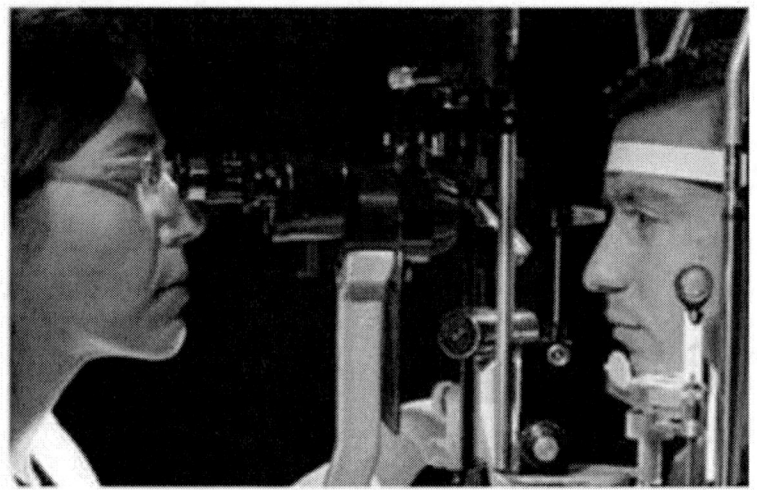

A tonometer measures pressure inside the eye to detect glaucoma.

Pachymetry is the measurement of the thickness of your cornea. Your eye care professional applies a numbing drop to your eye and uses an ultrasonic wave instrument to measure the thickness of your cornea.

Can Glaucoma Be Cured?

No. There is no cure for glaucoma. Vision lost from the disease cannot be restored.

Glaucoma Treatments

Immediate treatment for early-stage, open-angle glaucoma can delay progression of the disease. That's why early diagnosis is very important.

Glaucoma treatments include medicines, laser trabeculoplasty, conventional surgery, or a combination of any of these. While these treatments may save remaining vision, they do not improve sight already lost from glaucoma.

Medicines

Medicines, in the form of eyedrops or pills, are the most common early treatment for glaucoma. Taken regularly, these eyedrops lower eye pressure. Some medicines cause the eye to make less fluid. Others lower pressure by helping fluid drain from the eye.

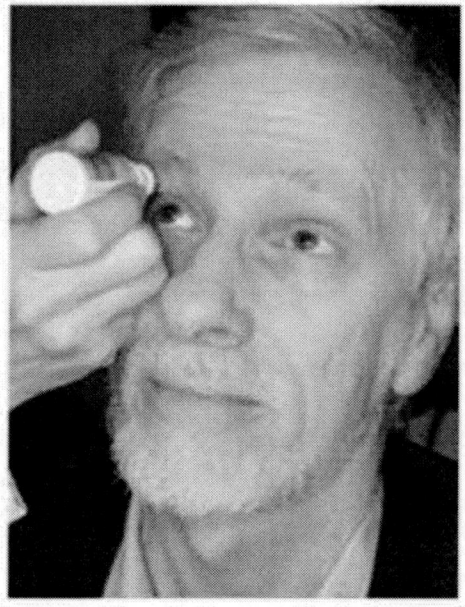

Before you begin glaucoma treatment, tell your eye care professional about other medicines and supplements that you are taking. Sometimes the drops can interfere with the way other medicines work.

Glaucoma medicines need to be taken regularly as directed by your eye care professional. Most people have no problems. However, some medicines can cause headaches or other side effects. For example, drops may cause stinging, burning, and redness in the eyes.

Many medicines are available to treat glaucoma. If you have problems with one medicine, tell your eye care professional. Treatment with a different dose or a new medicine may be possible.

Because glaucoma often has no symptoms, people may be tempted to stop taking, or may forget to take, their medicine. You need to use the drops or pills as long as they help control your eye pressure. Regular use is very important.

Make sure your eye care professional shows you how to put the drops into your eye. For tips on using your glaucoma eyedrops, see the end of this chapter.

Laser trabeculoplasty. Laser trabeculoplasty helps fluid drain out of the eye. Your doctor may suggest this step at any time. In many cases, you will need to keep taking glaucoma medicines after this procedure.

Laser trabeculoplasty is performed in your doctor's office or eye clinic. Before the surgery, numbing drops are applied to your eye. As you sit facing the laser machine, your doctor holds a special lens to your eye. A high-intensity beam of light is aimed through the lens and reflected onto the meshwork inside your eye. You may see flashes of bright green or red light. The laser makes several evenly spaced burns that stretch the drainage holes in the meshwork. This allows the fluid to drain better.

Like any surgery, laser surgery can cause side effects, such as inflammation. Your doctor may give you some drops to take home for any soreness or inflammation inside the eye. You will need to make several follow-up visits to have your eye pressure and eye monitored.

If you have glaucoma in both eyes, usually only one eye will be treated at a time. Laser treatments for each eye will be scheduled several days to several weeks apart.

Studies show that laser surgery can be very good at reducing the pressure in some patients. However, its effects can wear off over time. Your doctor may suggest further treatment.

Conventional Surgery

Conventional surgery makes a new opening for the fluid to leave the eye. (Diagram follows.) Your doctor may suggest this treatment at any time. Conventional surgery often is done after medicines and laser surgery have failed to control pressure.

Conventional surgery, called trabeculectomy, is performed in an operating room. Before the surgery, you are given medicine to help you relax. Your doctor makes small injections around the eye to numb it. A small piece of tissue is removed to create a new channel for the fluid to drain from the eye. This fluid will drain between the eye tissue layers and create a blister-like "filtration bleb." For several weeks after the surgery, you must put drops in the eye to fight infection and inflammation. These drops will be different from those you may have been using before surgery.

Conventional surgery is performed on one eye at a time. Usually the operations are four to six weeks apart.

Conventional surgery is about 60 to 80 percent effective at lowering eye pressure. If the new drainage opening narrows, a second operation may be needed. Conventional surgery works best if you have not had previous eye surgery, such as a cataract operation.

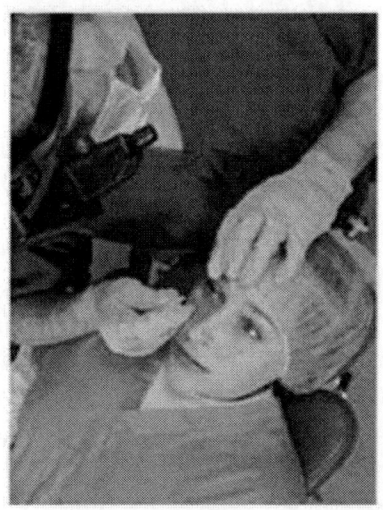

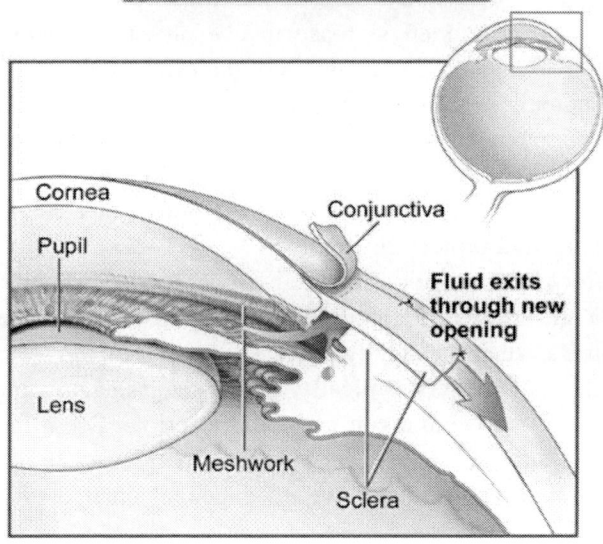

Sometimes after conventional surgery, your vision may not be as good as it was before conventional surgery. Conventional surgery can cause side effects, including cataract, problems with the cornea, inflammation, infection inside the eye, or low eye pressure problems. If you have any of these problems, tell your doctor so a treatment plan can be developed.

What Are Some Other Forms of Glaucoma?

Open-angle glaucoma is the most common form. Some people have other types of the disease.

In *low-tension* or *normal-tension glaucoma*, optic nerve damage and narrowed side vision occur in people with normal eye pressure. Lowering eye pressure at least 30 percent through medicines slows the disease in some people. Glaucoma may worsen in others despite low pressures.

A comprehensive medical history is important to identify other potential risk factors, such as low blood pressure, that contribute to low-tension glaucoma. If no risk factors are identified, the treatment options for low-tension glaucoma are the same as for open-angle glaucoma.

In *angle-closure glaucoma*, the fluid at the front of the eye cannot drain through the angle and leave the eye.

The angle gets blocked by part of the iris. People with this type of glaucoma may have a sudden increase in eye pressure. Symptoms include severe pain and nausea, as well as redness of the eye and blurred vision. If you have these symptoms, you need to seek treatment immediately. *This is a medical emergency*. If your doctor is unavailable, go to the nearest hospital or clinic. Without treatment to restore the flow of fluid, the eye can become blind. Usually, prompt laser surgery and medicines can clear the blockage, lower eye pressure, and protect vision.

In *congenital glaucoma*, children are born with a defect in the angle of the eye that slows the normal drainage of fluid. These children usually have obvious symptoms, such as cloudy eyes, sensitivity to light, and excessive tearing. Conventional surgery typically is the suggested treatment, because medicines are not effective and can cause more serious side effects in infants and be difficult to administer. Surgery is safe and effective. If surgery is done promptly, these children usually have an excellent chance of having good vision.

Secondary glaucomas can develop as complications of other medical conditions. For example, a severe form of glaucoma is called *neovascular glaucoma,* and can be a result from poorly controlled diabetes or high blood pressure. Other types of glaucoma sometimes occur with cataract, certain eye tumors, or when the eye is inflamed or irritated by a condition called uveitis. Sometimes glaucoma develops after other eye surgeries or serious eye injuries. Steroid drugs used to treat eye inflammations and other diseases can trigger glaucoma in some people. There are two eye conditions known to cause secondary forms of glaucoma. *Pigmentary glaucoma* occurs when pigment from the iris sheds off and blocks the meshwork, slowing fluid drainage. *Pseudoexfoliation glaucoma* occurs when extra material is produced and shed off internal eye structures and blocks the meshwork, again slowing fluid drainage.

Depending on the cause of these secondary glaucomas, treatment includes medicines, laser surgery, or conventional or other glaucoma surgery.

What Research Is Being Done?

Through studies in the laboratory and with patients, NEI is seeking better ways to detect, treat, and prevent vision loss in people with glaucoma. For example, researchers have discovered genes that could help explain how glaucoma damages the eye.

NEI also is supporting studies to learn more about who is likely to get glaucoma, when to treat people who have increased eye pressure, and which treatment to use first.

What You Can Do

If you are being treated for glaucoma, be sure to take your glaucoma medicine every day. See your eye care professional regularly.

You also can help protect the vision of family members and friends who may be at high risk for glaucoma—African Americans over age 40; everyone over age 60, especially Mexican Americans; and people with a family history of the disease. Encourage them to have a comprehensive dilated eye exam at least once every two years. Remember that lowering eye pressure in the early stages of glaucoma slows progression of the disease and helps save vision.

Medicare covers an annual comprehensive dilated eye exam for some people at high risk for glaucoma. These people include those with diabetes, those with a family history of glaucoma, and African Americans age 50 and older.

What Should I Ask My Eye Care Professional?

You can protect yourself against vision loss by working in partnership with your eye care professional. Ask questions and get the information you need to take care of yourself and your family.

What Are Some Questions to Ask?

About My Eye Disease or Disorder...
- What is my diagnosis?
- What caused my condition?
- Can my condition be treated?
- How will this condition affect my vision now and in the future?
- Should I watch for any particular symptoms and notify you if they occur?
- Should I make any lifestyle changes?

About My Treatment...
- What is the treatment for my condition?
- When will the treatment start and how long will it last?
- What are the benefits of this treatment and how successful is it?
- What are the risks and side effects associated with this treatment?
- Are there foods, medicines, or activities I should avoid while I'm on this treatment?
- If my treatment includes taking medicine, what should I do if I miss a dose?
- Are other treatments available?

About My Tests...
- What kinds of tests will I have?
- What can I expect to find out from these tests?

- When will I know the results?
- Do I have to do anything special to prepare for any of the tests?
- Do these tests have any side effects or risks?
- Will I need more tests later?

Other Suggestions
- If you don't understand your eye care professional's responses, ask questions until you do understand.
- Take notes or get a friend or family member to take notes for you. Or, bring a tape recorder to help you remember the discussion.
- Ask your eye care professional to write down his or her instructions to you.
- Ask your eye care professional for printed material about your condition.
- If you still have trouble understanding your eye care professional's answers, ask where you can go for more information.
- Other members of your healthcare team, such as nurses and pharmacists, can be good sources of information. Talk to them, too.

Today, patients take an active role in their health care. Be an active patient about your eye care.

Loss of Vision

If you have lost some sight from glaucoma, ask your eye care professional about low vision services and devices that may help you make the most of your remaining vision. Ask for a referral to a specialist in low vision. Many community organizations and agencies offer information about low vision counseling, training, and other special services for people with visual impairments.

Where Can I Get More Information?

For more information about glaucoma, contact the following organizations:

American Academy of Ophthalmology*
P.O. Box 7424
San Francisco, CA 94120–7424
415–561–8500
1–800–391–3937 (Eye Care America Glaucoma Project)
www.aao.org

American Optometric Association*
243 North Lindbergh Boulevard
St. Louis, MO 63141–7851
314–991–4100 www.aoa.org

The Glaucoma Foundation
80 Maiden Lane, Suite 1206
New York, NY 10038
212–285–0080
Email: info@glaucomafoundation.org
www.glaucoma-foundation.org/

Glaucoma Research Foundation
251 Post Street, Suite 600 San Francisco, CA 94108
1–800–826–6693
415–986–3162
www.glaucoma.org

National Eye Institute*
National Institutes of Health 2020 Vision Place
Bethesda, MD 20892–3655
301–496–5248
Email: 2020@nei.nih.gov
www.nei.nih.gov

Prevent Blindness America
211 West Wacker Drive, Suite 1700 Chicago, IL 60606
1–800–331–2020
312–363–6001
Email: info@preventblindness.org
www.preventblindness.org

*These organizations also provide information on low vision.

For more information about low vision services and programs, contact the following organizations:

American Foundation for the Blind
2 Penn Plaza, Suite 1102 New York, NY 10121
1–800–232–5463
212–502–7600
E-mail: afbinfo@afb.net
www.afb.org

Council of Citizens with Low Vision International
1–800–733–2258

Lighthouse International
111 East 59th Street
New York, NY 10022–1202
1–800–334–5497
1–800–829–0500
212–821–9200
212–821–9713 (TDD)
E-mail: info@lighthouse.org
www.lighthouse.org

How Should I Use My Glaucoma Eyedrops?

If eyedrops have been prescribed for treating your glaucoma, you need to use them properly, as instructed by your eye care professional. Proper use of your glaucoma medication can improve the medicine's effectiveness and reduce your risk of side effects.

To properly apply your eyedrops, follow these steps:

- Wash your hands.
- Hold the bottle upside down.
- Tilt your head back.
- Hold the bottle in one hand and place it as close as possible to the eye.

- With the other hand, pull down your lower eyelid. This forms a pocket.
- Place the prescribed number of drops into the lower eyelid pocket. If you are using more than one eyedrop, be sure to wait at least 5 minutes before applying the second eyedrop.

Close your eye OR press the lower lid lightly with your finger for at least 1 minute. Either of these steps keeps the drops in the eye and helps prevent the drops from draining into the tear duct, which can increase your risk of side effects.

The National Eye Institute (NEI) conducts and supports research that leads to sight-saving treatments and plays a key role in reducing visual impairment and blindness. NEI is part of the National Institutes of Health, an agency of the U.S. Department of Health and Human Services.

For more information, contact—

National Eye Institute
National Institutes of Health 2020 Vision Place
Bethesda, MD 20892–3655
Telephone: 301–496–5248
Email: 2020@nei.nih.gov
Website: www.nei.nih.gov

In: Eye Diseases and Disorders
Editor: Rachael Gray

ISBN: 978-1-63463-895-1
© 2015 Nova Science Publishers, Inc.

Chapter 2

Cataract: What You Should Know[*]

National Eye Institute

What Is a Cataract?

A cataract is a clouding of the lens in the eye that affects vision. Most cataracts are related to aging. Cataracts are very common in older people. By age 80, more than half of all Americans have either a cataract or have had cataract surgery.

A cataract can occur in either or both eyes. It cannot spread from one eye to the other.

What Is the Lens?

The lens is a clear part of the eye that helps to focus light, or an image, on the retina. The retina is the light-sensitive tissue at the back of the eye. (See diagram below.)

---

[*] This is an edited, reformatted and augmented version of a document (revised September 2014) issued by the National Institutes of Health, National Eye Institute.

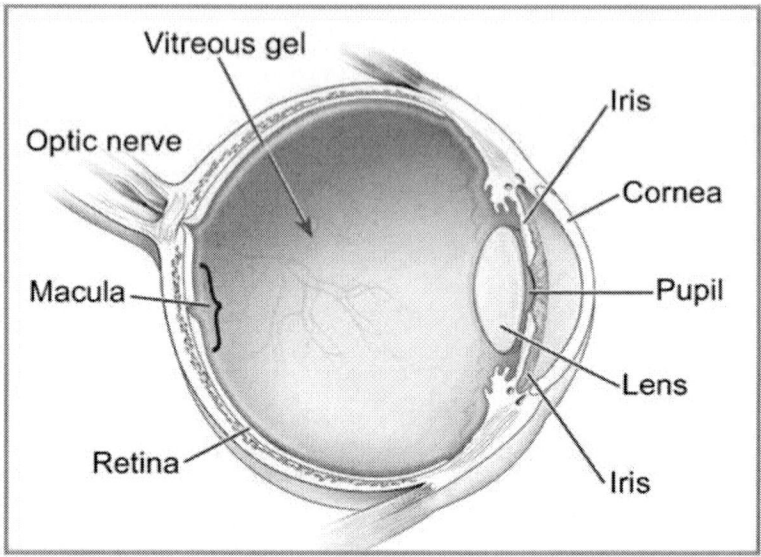

In a normal eye, light passes through the transparent lens to the retina. Once it reaches the retina, light is changed into nerve signals that are sent to the brain.

The lens must be clear for the retina to receive a sharp image. If the lens is cloudy from a cataract, the image you see will be blurred.

What Causes Cataracts?

The lens lies behind the iris and the pupil. It works much like a camera lens. It focuses light onto the retina at the back of the eye, where an image is recorded. The lens also adjusts the eye's focus, letting us see things clearly both up close and far away. The lens is made of mostly water and protein. The protein is arranged in a precise way that keeps the lens clear and lets light pass through it.

But as we age, some of the protein may clump together and start to cloud a small area of the lens. This is a cataract. Over time, the cataract may grow larger and cloud more of the lens, making it harder to see.

Smoking and diabetes contribute to the development of cataract. Or, it may be that the protein in the lens just changes from the wear and tear it takes over the years.

How Do Cataracts Affect Vision?

Age-related cataracts can affect vision in two ways:

1. Clumps of Protein Reduce the Sharpness of the Image Reaching the Retina

The lens consists mostly of water and protein. When the protein clumps up, it clouds the lens and reduces the light that reaches the retina. The clouding may become severe enough to cause blurred vision. Most age-related cataracts develop from protein clumpings.

When a cataract is small, the cloudiness affects only a small part of the lens. You may not notice any changes in your vision. Cataracts tend to "grow" slowly, so vision gets worse gradually. Over time, the cloudy area in the lens may get larger, and the cataract may increase in size. Seeing may become more difficult. Your vision may get duller or blurrier.

2. The Clear Lens Slowly Changes to a Yellowish/Brownish Color, Adding a Brownish Tint to Vision

As the clear lens slowly colors with age, your vision gradually may acquire a brownish shade. At first, the amount of tinting may be small and may not cause a vision problem. Over time, the cataract usually increases in size. This gradual change in the amount of tinting does not affect the sharpness of the image transmitted to the retina.

If you have advanced lens discoloration, you may not be able to identify blues and purples. You may be wearing what you believe to be a pair of black socks, only to find out from friends that you are wearing purple socks.

When Are You Most Likely to Have a Cataract?

The term "age-related" is a little misleading. You don't have to be a senior citizen to get this type of cataract. In fact, people can have an age-related cataract in their 40s and 50s. But during middle age, most cataracts are small and do not affect vision. It is after age 60 that most cataracts cause problems with a person's vision.

Who Is at Risk for Cataract?

The risk of cataract increases as you get older. Other risk factors for cataract include:

- Certain diseases (for example, diabetes).
- Personal behavior (smoking, alcohol use).
- The environment (prolonged exposure to ultraviolet sunlight).

What Are the Symptoms of a Cataract?

The most common symptoms of a cataract are:

- Cloudy or blurry vision.
- Colors seem faded.
- Glare. Headlights, lamps, or sunlight may appear too bright. A halo may appear around lights.
- Poor night vision.
- Double vision or multiple images in one eye. (This symptom may clear as the cataract gets larger.)
- Frequent prescription changes in your eyeglasses or contact lenses.

These symptoms also can be a sign of other eye problems. If you have any of these symptoms, check with your eye care professional.

Are There Different Types of Cataract?

Yes. Although most cataracts are related to aging, there are other types of cataract:

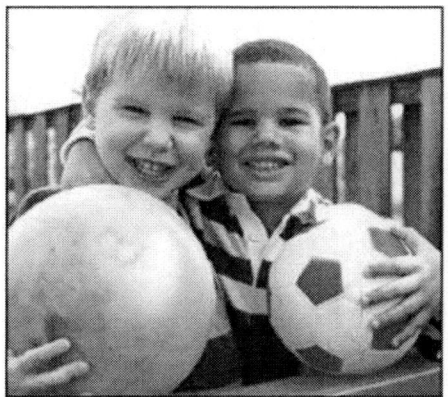
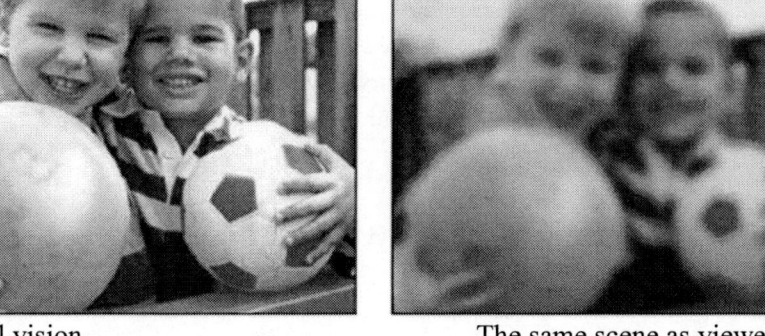

Normal vision   The same scene as viewed by a person with cataract

- *Secondary cataract.* Cataracts can form after surgery for other eye problems, such as glaucoma. Cataracts also can develop in people who have other health problems, such as diabetes. Cataracts are sometimes linked to steroid use.
- Traumatic cataract. Cataracts can develop after an eye injury, sometimes years later.
- Congenital cataract. Some babies are born with cataracts or develop them in childhood, often in both eyes. These cataracts may be so small that they do not affect vision. If they do, the lenses may need to be removed.
- Radiation cataract. Cataracts can develop after exposure to some types of radiation.

How Is a Cataract Detected?

Cataract is detected through a comprehensive eye exam that includes:

- Visual acuity test. This eye chart test measures how well you see at various distances.
- Dilated eye exam. Drops are placed in your eyes to widen, or dilate, the pupils. Your eye care professional uses a special magnifying lens to examine your retina and optic nerve for signs of damage and other

eye problems. After the exam, your close-up vision may remain blurred for several hours.
- Tonometry. An instrument measures the pressure inside the eye. Numbing drops may be applied to your eye for this test.
- Your eye care professional also may do other tests to learn more about the structure and health of your eye.

How Is a Cataract Treated?

The symptoms of early cataract may be improved with new eyeglasses, brighter lighting, anti-glare sunglasses, or magnifying lenses. If these measures do not help, surgery is the only effective treatment. Surgery involves removing the cloudy lens and replacing it with an artificial lens.

A cataract needs to be removed only when vision loss interferes with your everyday activities, such as driving, reading, or watching TV. You and your eye care professional can make this decision together. Once you understand the benefits and risks of surgery, you can make an informed decision about whether cataract surgery is right for you. In most cases, delaying cataract surgery will not cause long-term damage to your eye or make the surgery more difficult. You do not have to rush into surgery.

Sometimes a cataract should be removed even if it does not cause problems with your vision. For example, a cataract should be removed if it prevents examination or treatment of another eye problem, such as age-related macular degeneration or diabetic retinopathy.

If you choose surgery, your eye care professional may refer you to a specialist to remove the cataract.

If you have cataracts in both eyes that require surgery, the surgery will be performed on each eye at separate times, usually four weeks apart.

Is Cataract Surgery Effective?

Cataract removal is one of the most common operations performed in the United States. It also is one of the safest and most effective types of surgery. In about 90 percent of cases, people who have cataract surgery have better vision afterward.

What Are the Risks of Cataract Surgery?

As with any surgery, cataract surgery poses risks, such as infection and bleeding. Before cataract surgery, your doctor may ask you to temporarily stop taking certain medications that increase the risk of bleeding during surgery. After surgery, you must keep your eye clean, wash your hands before touching your eye, and use the prescribed medications to help minimize the risk of infection. Serious infection can result in loss of vision.

Cataract surgery slightly increases your risk of retinal detachment. Other eye disorders, such as high myopia (nearsightedness), can further increase your risk of retinal detachment after cataract surgery. One sign of a retinal detachment is a sudden increase in flashes or floaters. Floaters are little "cobwebs" or specks that seem to float about in your field of vision. If you notice a sudden increase in floaters or flashes, see an eye care professional immediately. A retinal detachment is a medical emergency. If necessary, go to an emergency service or hospital. Your eye must be examined by a physician as soon as possible. A retinal detachment causes no pain. Early treatment for retinal detachment often can prevent permanent loss of vision. The longer the retina stays detached, the less likely you will regain good vision once you are treated. Even if you are treated promptly, some vision may be lost.

Talk to your eye care professional about these risks. Make sure cataract surgery is right for you.

What if I Have Other Eye Conditions and Need Cataract Surgery?

Many people who need cataract surgery also have other eye conditions, such as age-related macular degeneration or glaucoma. If you have other eye conditions in addition to cataract, talk with your doctor. Learn about the risks, benefits, alternatives, and expected results of cataract surgery.

What Happens before Surgery?

A week or two before surgery, your doctor will do some tests. These tests may include measuring the curve of the cornea and the size and shape of your eye. This information helps your doctor choose the right type of IOL.

You may be asked not to eat or drink anything 12 hours before your surgery.

What Happens during Surgery?

At the hospital or eye clinic, drops will be put into your eye to dilate the pupil. The area around your eye will be washed and cleansed.

The operation usually lasts less than one hour and is almost painless. Many people choose to stay awake during surgery. Others may need to be put to sleep for a short time. If you are awake, you will have an anesthetic to numb your eye.

After the operation, a patch may be placed over your eye. You will rest for a while. Your medical team will watch for any problems, such as bleeding. Most people who have cataract surgery can go home the same day. You will need someone to drive you home.

What Happens after Surgery?

Itching and mild discomfort are normal after cataract surgery. Some fluid discharge is also common. Your eye may be sensitive to light and touch. If you have discomfort, your doctor can suggest treatment. After one or two days, moderate discomfort should disappear.

For a few weeks after surgery, your doctor may ask you to use eyedrops to help healing and decrease the risk of infection. Ask your doctor about how to use your eyedrops, how often to use them, and what effects they can have. You will need to wear an eye shield or eyeglasses to help protect your eye. Avoid rubbing or pressing on your eye.

When you are home, try not to bend from the waist to pick up objects on the floor. Do not lift any heavy objects. You can walk, climb stairs, and do light household chores.

In most cases, healing will be complete within eight weeks. Your doctor will schedule exams to check on your progress.

Can Problems Develop after Surgery?

Problems after surgery are rare, but they can occur. These problems can include infection, bleeding, inflammation (pain, redness, swelling), loss of vision, double vision, and high or low eye pressure. With prompt medical attention, these problems usually can be treated successfully.

Sometimes the eye tissue that encloses the IOL becomes cloudy and may blur your vision. This condition is called an after-cataract. An after-cataract can develop months or years after cataract surgery.

An after-cataract is treated with a laser. Your doctor uses a laser to make a tiny hole in the eye tissue behind the lens to let light pass through. This outpatient procedure is called a YAG laser capsulotomy. It is painless and rarely results in increased eye pressure or other eye problems. As a precaution, your doctor may give you eyedrops to lower your eye pressure before or after the procedure.

When Will My Vision Be Normal Again?

You can return quickly to many everyday activities, but your vision may be blurry. The healing eye needs time to adjust so that it can focus properly with the other eye, especially if the other eye has a cataract. Ask your doctor when you can resume driving.

If you received an IOL, you may notice that colors are very bright. Most IOLs are clear, unlike your natural lens that may have had a yellowish/brownish tint. Within a few months after receiving an IOL, you will become used to improved color vision. Also, when your eye heals, you will most likely need new glasses or contact lenses.

What Can I Do if I Already Have Lost Some Vision from Cataract?

If you have lost some vision, speak with your surgeon about options that may help you make the most of your remaining vision.

What Research Is Being Done?

The National Eye Institute is conducting and supporting a number of studies focusing on factors associated with the development of age-related cataract. These studies include:

- The effect of sunlight exposure, which may be associated with an increased risk of cataract.
- Vitamin supplements, which have shown varying results in delaying the progression of cataract.
- Genetic studies, which show promise for better understanding cataract development.

What Can I Do to Protect My Vision?

Wearing sunglasses and a hat with a brim to block ultraviolet sunlight may help to delay cataract. If you smoke, stop. Researchers also believe good nutrition can help reduce the risk of age-related cataract. They recommend eating green leafy vegetables, fruit, and other foods with antioxidants.

If you are age 60 or older, you should have a comprehensive dilated eye exam at least once every two years. In addition to cataract, your eye care professional can check for signs of age-related macular degeneration, glaucoma, and other vision disorders. Early treatment for many eye diseases may save your sight.

What Should I Ask My Eye Care Professional?

You can protect yourself against vision loss by working in partnership with your eye care professional. Ask questions and get the information you need to take care of yourself and your family.

What Are Some Questions to Ask?

About my eye disease or disorder...

- What is my diagnosis?
- What caused my condition?
- Can my condition be treated?
- How will this condition affect my vision now and in the future?
- Should I watch for any particular symptoms and notify you if they occur?
- Should I make any lifestyle changes?

About my treatment...

- What is the treatment for my condition?
- When will the treatment start and how long will it last?
- What are the benefits of this treatment and how successful is it?
- What are the risks and side effects associated with this treatment?
- Are there foods, drugs, or activities I should avoid while I'm on this treatment?
- If my treatment includes taking medicine, what should I do if I miss a dose?
- Are other treatments available?

About my tests...

- What kinds of tests will I have?
- What can I expect to find out from these tests?
- When will I know the results?
- Do I have to do anything special to prepare for any of the tests?
- Do these tests have any side effects or risks?
- Will I need more tests later?

Other suggestions

- If you don't understand your eye care professional's responses, ask questions until you do understand.

- Take notes or get a friend or family member to take notes for you. Or, bring a tape recorder to help you remember the discussion.
- Ask your eye care professional to write down his or her instructions to you.
- Ask your eye care professional for printed material about your condition.
- If you still have trouble understanding your eye care professional's answers, ask where you can go for more information.
- Other members of your health care team, such as nurses and pharmacists, can be good sources of information. Talk to them, too.

Today, patients take an active role in their health care. Be an active patient about your eye care.

Where Can I Get More Information?

For more information about cataract, you may wish to contact:

American Academy of Ophthalmology*
P.O. Box 7424
San Francisco, CA 94109–7424
415–561–8500
www.aao.org

American Optometric Association*
243 North Lindbergh Boulevard
St. Louis, MO 63141–7851
314–991–4100
www.aoa.org

National Eye Institute*
National Institutes of Health
2020 Vision Place
Bethesda, MD 20892–3655
301–496–5248
Email: 2020@nei.nih.gov
www.nei.nih.gov

Prevent Blindness America
211 West Wacker Drive, 17th Floor
Chicago, IL 60606
1–800–331–2020, ext. 6026
312–363–6026
Email: info@preventblindness.org
www.preventblindness.org

* These organizations also provide information on low vision.

For more information about IOLs, contact:
U.S. Food and Drug Administration
Office of Consumer Affairs Parklawn Building (HFE–88)
5600 Fishers Lane
Rockville, MD 20857
1–888–463–6332
www.fda.gov

In: Eye Diseases and Disorders
Editor: Rachael Gray

ISBN: 978-1-63463-895-1
© 2015 Nova Science Publishers, Inc.

Chapter 3

Age-Related Macular Degeneration: What You Should Know[*]

National Eye Institute

What You Should Know About Age-Related Macular Degeneration (AMD)

Perhaps you have just learned that you or a loved one has age-related macular degeneration, also known as AMD. If you are like many people, you probably do not know a lot about the condition or understand what is going on inside your eyes.

This chapter will give you a general overview of AMD. You will learn about the following:

- Risk factors and symptoms of AMD
- Treatment options
- Low vision services that help people make the most of their remaining eyesight
- Support groups and others who can help

---

[*] This is an edited, reformatted and augmented version of a document (revised September 2014) issued by the National Institutes of Health, National Eye Institute.

The aim is to answer your questions and to help relieve some of the anxiety you may be feeling.

What is AMD?

AMD is a common eye condition and a leading cause of vision loss among people age 60 and older. It causes damage to the macula, a small spot near the center of the retina and the part of the eye needed for sharp, central vision, which lets us see objects that are straight ahead.

In some people, AMD advances so slowly that vision loss does not occur for a long time. In others, the disease progresses faster and may lead to a loss of vision in one or both eyes. As AMD progresses, a blurred area near the center of vision is a common symptom. Over time, the blurred area may grow larger or you may develop blank spots in your central vision. Objects also may not appear to be as bright as they used to be.

AMD by itself does not lead to complete blindness, with no ability to see. However, the loss of central vision in AMD can interfere with simple everyday activities, such as the ability to see faces, drive, read, write, or do close work, such as cooking or fixing things around the house.

The Macula

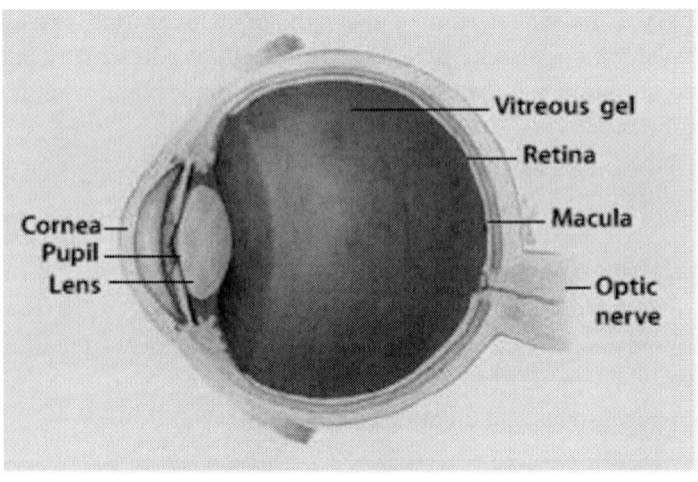

The macula is made up of millions of light-sensing cells that provide sharp, central vision. It is the most sensitive part of the retina, which is located at the back of the eye. The retina turns light into electrical signals and then sends these electrical signals through the optic nerve to the brain, where they are translated into the images we see. When the macula is damaged, the center of your field of view may appear blurry, distorted, or dark.

Who Is at Risk?

Age is a major risk factor for AMD. The disease is most likely to occur after age 60, but it can occur earlier. Other risk factors for AMD include:

- Smoking. Research shows that smoking doubles the risk of AMD.
- Race. AMD is more common among Caucasians than among African-Americans or Hispanics/Latinos.
- Family history. People with a family history of AMD are at higher risk.

Does Lifestyle Make a Difference?

Researchers have found links between AMD and some lifestyle choices, such as smoking. You might be able to reduce your risk of AMD or slow its progression by making these healthy choices:

- Avoid smoking
- Exercise regularly
- Maintain normal blood pressure and cholesterol levels
- Eat a healthy diet rich in green, leafy vegetables and fish

How Is AMD Detected?

The early and intermediate stages of AMD usually start without symptoms. Only a comprehensive dilated eye exam can detect AMD. The eye exam may include the following:

- Visual acuity test. This eye chart measures how well you see at distances.
- Dilated eye exam. Your eye care professional places drops in your eyes to widen or dilate the pupils. This provides a better view of the back of your eye. Using a special magnifying lens, he or she then looks at your retina and optic nerve for signs of AMD and other eye problems.
- Amsler grid. Your eye care professional also may ask you to look at an Amsler grid. Changes in your central vision may cause the lines in the grid to disappear or appear wavy, a sign of AMD.

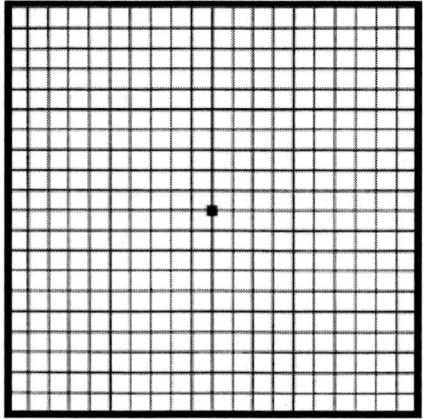

Here is what an Amsler grid normally looks like.

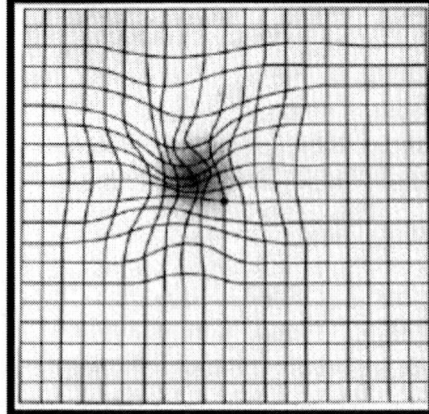

This is what an Amsler grid might look like to someone with AMD.

- Fluorescein angiogram. In this test, which is performed by an ophthalmologist, a fluorescent dye is injected into your arm. Pictures are taken as the dye passes through the blood vessels in your eye. This makes it possible to see leaking blood vessels, which occur in a severe, rapidly progressive type of AMD (see below). In rare cases, complications to the injection can arise, from nausea to more severe allergic reactions.
- Optical coherence tomography. You have probably heard of ultrasound, which uses sound waves to capture images of living tissues. OCT is similar except that it uses light waves, and can achieve very high-resolution images of any tissues that can be penetrated by light—such as the eyes. After your eyes are dilated, you'll be asked to place your head on a chin rest and hold still for several seconds while the images are obtained. The light beam is painless.
- During the exam, your eye care professional will look for drusen, which are yellow deposits beneath the retina. Most people develop some very small drusen as a normal part of aging. The presence of medium-to-large drusen may indicate that you have AMD.

Another sign of AMD is the appearance of pigmentary changes under the retina. In addition to the pigmented cells in the iris (the colored part of the eye), there are pigmented cells beneath the retina. As these cells break down and release their pigment, your eye care professional may see dark clumps of released pigment and later, areas that are less pigmented. These changes will not affect your eye color.

Questions to Ask Your Eye Care Professional

Below are a few questions you may want to ask your eye care professional to help you understand your diagnosis and treatment. If you do not understand your eye care professional's responses, ask questions until you do understand.

- What is my diagnosis and how do you spell the name of the condition?
- Can my AMD be treated?
- How will this condition affect my vision now and in the future?

- What symptoms should I watch for and how should I notify you if they occur?
- Should I make lifestyle changes?

What Are the Stages of AMD?

There are three stages of AMD defined in part by the size and number of drusen under the retina. It is possible to have AMD in one eye only, or to have one eye with a later stage of AMD than the other.

- Early AMD. Early AMD is diagnosed by the presence of medium-sized drusen, which are about the width of an average human hair. People with early AMD typically do not have vision loss.
- Intermediate AMD. People with intermediate AMD typically have large drusen, pigment changes in the retina, or both. Again, these changes can only be detected during an eye exam. Intermediate AMD may cause some vision loss, but most people will not experience any symptoms.
- Late AMD. In addition to drusen, people with late AMD have vision loss from damage to the macula. There are two types of late AMD:
- In geographic atrophy (also called dry AMD), there is a gradual breakdown of the light-sensitive cells in the macula that convey visual information to the brain, and of the supporting tissue beneath the macula. These changes cause vision loss.
- In neovascular AMD (also called wet AMD), abnormal blood vessels grow underneath the retina. ("Neovascular" literally means "new vessels.") These vessels can leak fluid and blood, which may lead to swelling and damage of the macula. The damage may be rapid and severe, unlike the more gradual course of geographic atrophy. It is possible to have both geographic atrophy and neovascular AMD in the same eye, and either condition can appear first.

AMD has few symptoms in the early stages, so it is important to have your eyes examined regularly. If you are at risk for AMD because of age, family history, lifestyle, or some combination of these factors, you should not wait to experience changes in vision before getting checked for AMD.

Not everyone with early AMD will develop late AMD. For people who have early AMD in one eye and no signs of AMD in the other eye, about five percent will develop advanced AMD after 10 years. For people who have early AMD in both eyes, about 14 percent will develop late AMD in at least one eye after 10 years. With prompt detection of AMD, there are steps you can take to further reduce your risk of vision loss from late AMD.

If you have late AMD in one eye only, you may not notice any changes in your overall vision. With the other eye seeing clearly, you may still be able to drive, read, and see fine details. However, having late AMD in one eye means you are at increased risk for late AMD in your other eye.

If you notice distortion or blurred vision, even if it doesn't have much effect on your daily life, consult an eye care professional.

How Is AMD Treated?

Early AMD

Currently, no treatment exists for early AMD, which in many people shows no symptoms or loss of vision. Your eye care professional may recommend that you get a comprehensive dilated eye exam at least once a year. The exam will help determine if your condition is advancing.

As for prevention, AMD occurs less often in people who exercise, avoid smoking, and eat nutritious foods including green leafy vegetables and fish. If you already have AMD, adopting some of these habits may help you keep your vision longer.

Intermediate and Late AMD

Researchers at the National Eye Institute tested whether taking nutritional supplements could protect against AMD in the Age-Related Eye Disease Studies (AREDS and AREDS2). They found that daily intake of certain high-dose vitamins and minerals can slow progression of the disease in people who have intermediate AMD, and those who have late AMD in one eye.

The first AREDS trial showed that a combination of vitamin C, vitamin E, beta-carotene, zinc, and copper can reduce the risk of late AMD by 25 percent. The AREDS2 trial tested whether this formulation could be improved by adding lutein, zeaxanthin or omega-3 fatty acids. Omega-3 fatty acids are nutrients enriched in fish oils. Lutein, zeaxanthin and beta-carotene all belong to the same family of vitamins, and are abundant in green leafy vegetables.

The AREDS2 trial found that adding lutein and zeaxanthin or omega-3 fatty acids to the original AREDS formulation (with beta-carotene) had no overall effect on the risk of late AMD. However, the trial also found that replacing beta-carotene with a 5-to-i mixture of lutein and zeaxanthin may help further reduce the risk of late AMD. Moreover, while beta-carotene has been linked to an increased risk of lung cancer in current and former smokers, lutein and zeaxanthin appear to be safe regardless of smoking status.

Here are the clinically effective doses tested in AREDS and AREDS2:

- 500 milligrams (mg) of vitamin C
- 400 international units of vitamin E
- 80 mg zinc as zinc oxide (25 mg in AREDS2)
- 2 mg copper as cupric oxide
- 15 mg beta-carotene, OR 10 mg lutein and 2 mg zeaxanthin

A number of manufacturers offer nutritional supplements that were formulated based on these studies. The label may refer to "AREDS" or "AREDS2."

If you have intermediate or late AMD, you might benefit from taking such supplements. But first, be sure to review and compare the labels. Many of the supplements have different ingredients, or different doses, from those tested in the AREDS trials. Also, consult your doctor or eye care professional about which supplement, if any, is right for you. For example, if you smoke regularly, or used to, your doctor may recommend that you avoid supplements containing beta-carotene.

Even if you take a daily multivitamin, you should consider taking an AREDS supplement if you are at risk for late AMD. The formulations tested in the AREDS trials contain much higher doses of vitamins and minerals than what is found in multivitamins. Tell your doctor or eye care professional about any multivitamins you are taking when you are discussing possible AREDS formulations.

Finally, remember that the AREDS formulation is not a cure. It does not help people with early AMD, and will not restore vision already lost from AMD. But it may delay the onset of late AMD. It also may help slow vision loss in people who already have late AMD.

Advanced Neovascular AMD

Neovascular AMD typically results in severe vision loss. However, eye care professionals can try different therapies to stop further vision loss. You should remember that the therapies described below are not a cure. The condition may progress even with treatment.

- Injections. One option to slow the progression of neovascular AMD is to inject drugs into the eye. With neovascular AMD, abnormally high levels of vascular endothelial growth factor (VEGF) are secreted in your eyes. VEGF is a protein that promotes the growth of new abnormal blood vessels. Anti-VEGF injection therapy blocks this growth. If you get this treatment, you may need multiple monthly injections. Before each injection, your eye will be numbed and cleaned with antiseptics. To further reduce the risk of infection, you may be prescribed antibiotic drops. A few different anti-VEGF drugs are available. They vary in cost and in how often they need to be injected, so you may wish to discuss these issues with your eye care professional.
- Photodynamic therapy. This technique involves laser treatment of select areas of the retina. First, a drug called verteporfin will be injected into a vein in your arm. The drug travels through the blood vessels in your body, and is absorbed by new, growing blood vessels. Your eye care professional then shines a laser beam into your eye to activate the drug in the new abnormal blood vessels, while sparing normal ones. Once activated, the drug closes off the new blood vessels, slows their growth, and slows the rate of vision loss. This procedure is less common than anti-VEGF injections, and is often used in combination with them for specific types of neovascular AMD.
- Laser surgery. Eye care professionals treat certain cases of neovascular AMD with laser surgery, though this is less common than other treatments. It involves aiming an intense "hot" laser at the abnormal blood vessels in your eyes to destroy them. This laser is not the same one used in photodynamic therapy which may be referred to as a "cold" laser. This treatment is more likely to be used when blood vessel growth is limited to a compact area in your eye, away from the center of the macula, that can be easily targeted with the laser. Even so, laser treatment also may destroy some surrounding healthy tissue.

This often results in a small blind spot where the laser has scarred the retina. In some cases, vision immediately after the surgery may be worse than it was before. But the surgery may also help prevent more severe vision loss from occurring years later.

Questions to Ask Your Eye Care Professional About Treatment

- What is the treatment for advanced neovascular AMD?
- When will treatment start and how long will it last?
- What are the benefits of this treatment and how successful is it?
- What are the risks and side effects associated with this treatment and how has this information been gathered?
- Should I avoid certain foods, drugs, or activities while I am undergoing treatment?
- Are other treatments available?
- When should I follow up after treatment?

How Can I Cope with Vision Loss?

Coping with AMD and vision loss can be a traumatic experience. This is especially true if you have just begun to lose your vision or have low vision. Having low vision means that even with regular glasses, contact lenses, medicine, or surgery, you find everyday tasks difficult to do. Reading the mail, shopping, cooking, and writing can all seem challenging.

However, help is available. You may not be able to restore your vision, but low vision services can help you make the most of what is remaining. You can continue enjoying friends, family, hobbies, and other interests just as you always have. The key is to not delay use of these services.

What Is Vision Rehabilitation?

To cope with vision loss, you must first have an excellent support team. This team should include you, your primary eye care professional, and an optometrist or ophthalmologist specializing in low vision. Occupational therapists, orientation and mobility specialists, certified low vision therapists, counselors, and social workers are also available to help. Together, the low vision team can help you make the most of your remaining vision and maintain your independence.

Second, talk with your eye care professional about your vision problems. Ask about vision rehabilitation, even if your eye care professional says that "nothing more can be done for your vision." Vision rehabilitation programs offer a wide range of services, including training for magnifying and adaptive devices, ways to complete daily living skills safely and independently, guidance on modifying your home, and information on where to locate resources and support to help you cope with your vision loss.

Medicare may cover part or all of a patient's occupational therapy, but the therapy must be ordered by a doctor and provided by a Medicare-approved healthcare provider. To see if you are eligible for Medicare-funded occupational therapy, call 1-800-MEDICARE or 1-800-633-4227.

Where Can I Go for Services?

Low vision services can take place in different locations, including:

- Ophthalmology or optometry offices that specialize in low vision
- Hospital clinics
- State, nonprofit, or for-profit vision rehabilitation organizations
- Independent-living centers

What Are Some Low Vision Devices?

Because low vision varies from person to person, specialists have different tools to help patients deal with vision loss. They include:

- Reading glasses with high-powered lenses
- Handheld magnifiers
- Video magnifiers
- Computers with large-print and speech-output systems
- Large-print reading materials
- Talking watches, clocks, and calculators

- Computer aids and other technologies, such as a closed-circuit television, which uses a camera and television to enlarge printed text

Keep in mind that low vision aids without proper diagnosis, evaluation, and training may not work for you. It is important that you work closely with your low vision team to get the best device or combination of aids to help improve your ability to see.

Questions to Ask Your Eye Care Professional About Low Vision

- How can I continue my normal, routine activities?
- Are there resources to help me?
- Will any special devices help me with reading, cooking, or fixing things around the house?
- What training is available to me?
- Where can I find individual or group support to cope with my vision loss?

What Is Charles Bonnet Syndrome (Visual Hallucinations)?

People with impaired vision sometimes see things that are not there, called visual hallucinations. They may see simple patterns of colors or shapes, or detailed pictures of people, animals, buildings, or landscapes. Sometimes these images fit logically into a visual scene, but they often do not.

This condition can be alarming, but don't worry—it is not a sign of mental illness. It is called Charles Bonnet syndrome, and it is similar to what happens to some people who have lost an arm or leg. Even though the limb is gone, these people still feel their toes or fingers or experience itching. Similarly, when the brain loses input from the eyes, it may fill the void by generating visual images on its own.

Charles Bonnet syndrome is a common side effect of vision loss in people with AMD. However, it often goes away a year to 18 months after it begins. In the meantime, there are things you can do to reduce hallucinations. Many people find the hallucinations occur more frequently in evening or dim light.

Turning on a light or television may help. It may also help to blink, close your eyes, or focus on a real object for a few moments.

How Can I Cope with AMD?

AMD and vision loss can profoundly affect your life. This is especially true if you lose your vision rapidly.

Even if you experience gradual vision loss, you may not be able to live your life the way you used to. You may need to cut back on working, volunteering, and recreational activities. Your relationships may change, and you may need more help from family and friends than you are used to. These changes can lead to feelings of loss, lowered self-esteem, isolation, and depression.

In addition to getting medical treatment for AMD, there are things you can do to cope:

- Learn more about your vision loss.
- Visit a specialist in low vision and get devices and learning skills to help you with the tasks of everyday living.
- Try to stay positive. People who remain hopeful say they are better able to cope with AMD and vision loss.
- Stay engaged with family and friends.
- Seek a professional counselor or support group. Your doctor or eye care professional may be able to refer you to one.

What Information Can I Share with Family Members?

Shock, disbelief, depression, and anger are common reactions among people who are diagnosed with AMD. These feelings can subside after a few days or weeks, or they may last longer. This can be upsetting to family members and caregivers who are trying to be as caring and supportive as possible.

Following are some ideas family members might consider:

- Obtain as much information as possible about AMD and how it affects sight. Share the information with the person who has AMD.
- Find support groups and other resources within the community.

- Encourage family and friends to visit and support the person with AMD.
- Allow for grieving. This is a natural process.
- Lend support by "being there."

Where Can I Get More Information?

For more information about age-related macular degeneration, you may wish to contact:

AMD Alliance International
1929 Bayview Avenue
Toronto, Ontario, Canada M4G 3E8
877-AMD-7171
416-486-2500 ext. 7505
E-mail: info@amdalliance.org
www.amdalliance.org

American Academy of Ophthalmology*
P.O. Box 7424
San Francisco, CA 94120–7424
415–561–8500
www.aao.org

American Foundation for the Blind ii Penn Plaza,
Suite 300 New York, NY 10011–2006 1-800-232-5463
212–502–7600
E-mail: afbinfo@afb.net
www.afb.org

American Optometric Association*
243 North Lindbergh Boulevard
St. Louis, MO 63141-7851
314-991-4100
www.aoa.org

Association for Macular Diseases
210 East 64th Street, 8th Floor New York, NY 10021–7471
212-605-3719
www.macular.org

Council of Citizens with Low Vision International
1-800-733-2258
www.cclvi.org

EyeCare America
P.O. Box 429098
San Francisco, CA 94142-0998 877-887-6327
E-mail: pubserv@aao.org
www.eyecareamerica.org

The Foundation Fighting Blindness
11435 Cronhill Drive
Owings Mill, MD 21117-2220
1-800-683-555
410–568–0150
800-683-5551 (TDD)
E-mail: info@fightblindness.org
www.blindness.org

Lighthouse International
111 East 59th Street
New York, NY 10022–1202
1-800-334-5497
1–800–829–0500
212–821–9200
212-821-9713 (TDD)
E-mail: info@lighthouse.org
www.lighthouse.org

Macular Degeneration Partnership
8733 Beverly Boulevard, Suite 201 Los Angeles,
CA 90048–1844 1-888-430-9898
310-423-6455
www.amd.org

National Eye Institute*
National Institutes of Health
2020 Vision Place
Bethesda, MD 20892-3655
301-496-5248
E-mail: 2020@nei.nih.gov
www.nei.nih.gov

Prevent Blindness America
211 West Wacker Drive, Suite 1700
Chicago, IL 60606
1-800-331-2020, ext. 6026
312-363-6026
E-mail: info@preventblindness.org
www.preventblindness.org

VisionAware*
http://www.visionaware.org

*These organizations also provide information on low vision.

In: Eye Diseases and Disorders
Editor: Rachael Gray

ISBN: 978-1-63463-895-1
© 2015 Nova Science Publishers, Inc.

Chapter 4

Diabetic Retinopathy: What You Should Know[*]

National Eye Institute

What Is Diabetic Retinopathy?

Diabetic retinopathy is a complication of diabetes and a leading cause of blindness. It occurs when diabetes damages the tiny blood vessels inside the retina, the light-sensitive tissue at the back of the eye. (See diagram on next page.) A healthy retina is necessary for good vision.

If you have diabetic retinopathy, at first you may notice no changes to your vision. But over time, diabetic retinopathy can get worse and cause vision loss. Diabetic retinopathy usually affects both eyes.

What Are the Stages of Diabetic Retinopathy?

Diabetic retinopathy has four stages:

---

[*] This is an edited, reformatted and augmented version of NIH Publication No: 06-2171, issued by the National Institutes of Health, National Eye Institute, September 2003.

1. Mild Nonproliferative Retinopathy. At this earliest stage, microaneurysms occur. They are small areas of balloon-like swelling in the retina's tiny blood vessels.
2. Moderate Nonproliferative Retinopathy. As the disease progresses, some blood vessels that nourish the retina are blocked.
3. Severe Nonproliferative Retinopathy. Many more blood vessels are blocked, depriving several areas of the retina with their blood supply. These areas of the retina send signals to the body to grow new blood vessels for nourishment.
4. Proliferative Retinopathy. At this advanced stage, the signals sent by the retina for nourishment trigger the growth of new blood vessels. This condition is called proliferative retinopathy. These new blood vessels are abnormal and fragile. They grow along the retina and along the surface of the clear, vitreous gel that fills the inside of the eye. (See diagram on below.)
5. By themselves, these blood vessels do not cause symptoms or vision loss. However, they have thin, fragile walls. If they leak blood, severe vision loss and even blindness can result.

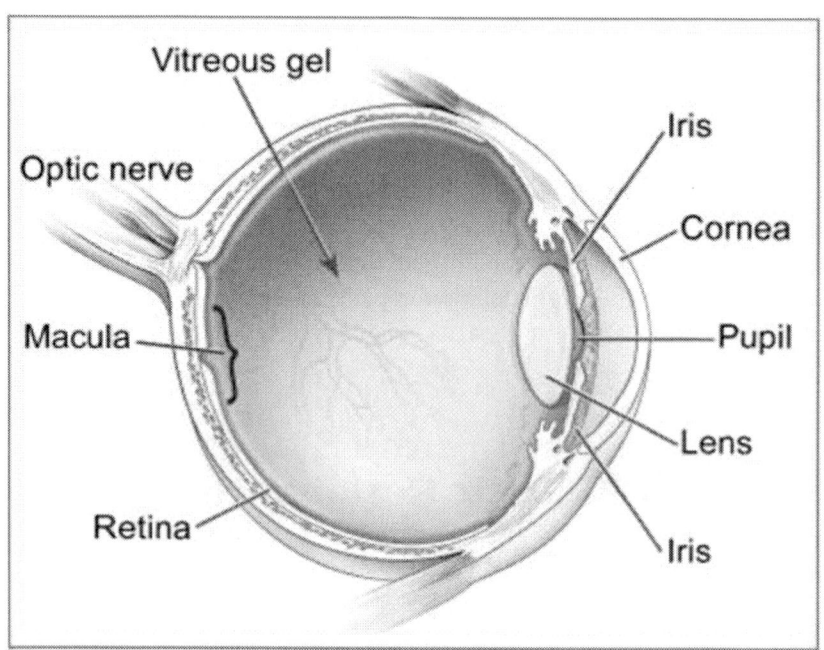

Who Is at Risk for Diabetic Retinopathy?

All people with diabetes—both type 1 and type 2—are at risk. That's why everyone with diabetes should get a comprehensive dilated eye exam at least once a year. Between 40 to 45 percent of Americans diagnosed with diabetes have some stage of diabetic retinopathy. If you have diabetic retinopathy, your doctor can recommend treatment to help prevent its progression.

During pregnancy, diabetic retinopathy may be a problem for women with diabetes. To protect vision, *every* pregnant woman with diabetes should have a comprehensive dilated eye exam as soon as possible. Your doctor may recommend additional exams during your pregnancy.

How Does Diabetic Retinopathy Cause Vision Loss?

Blood vessels damaged from diabetic retinopathy can cause vision loss in two ways:

1. Fragile, abnormal blood vessels can develop and leak blood into the center of the eye, blurring vision. This is proliferative retinopathy and is the fourth and most advanced stage of the disease.
2. Fluid can leak into the center of the macula, the part of the eye where sharp, straight-ahead vision occurs. The fluid makes the macula swell, blurring vision. This condition is called macular edema. It can occur at any stage of diabetic retinopathy, although it is more likely to occur as the disease progresses. About half of the people with proliferative retinopathy also have macular edema.

Does Diabetic Retinopathy Have Any Symptoms?

Diabetic retinopathy often has no early warning signs. Don't wait for symptoms. Be sure to have a comprehensive dilated eye exam at least once a year.

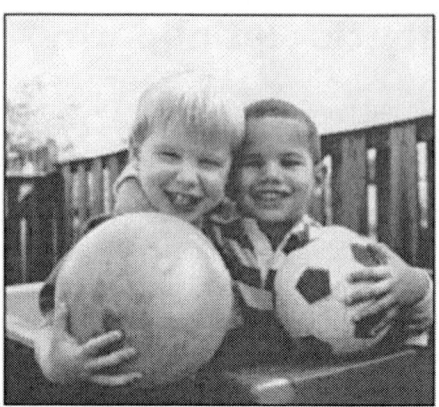
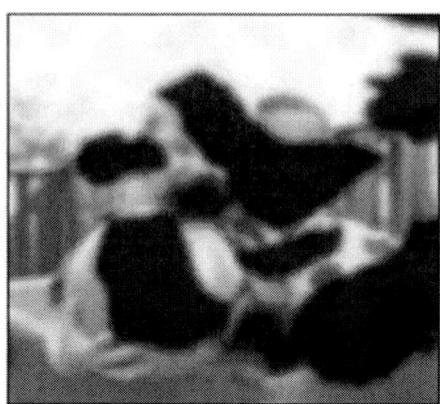

Normal vision

Same scene viewed by a person with diabetic retinopathy

What Are the Symptoms of Proliferative Retinopathy if Bleeding Occurs?

At first, you will see a few specks of blood, or spots, "floating" in your vision. If spots occur, see your eye care professional as soonas possible. You may need treatment before more serious bleeding occurs. Hemorrhages tend to happen more than once, often during sleep.

Sometimes, without treatment, the spots clear, and you will see better. However, bleeding can reoccur and cause severely blurred vision. You need to be examined by your eye care professional at the first sign of blurred vision, before more bleeding occurs.

If left untreated, proliferative retinopathy can cause severe vision loss and even blindness. Also, the earlier you receive treatment, the more likely treatment will be effective.

How Are Macular Edema and Diabetic Retinopathy Detected?

Macular edema and diabetic retinopathy are detected during a comprehensive eye exam that includes:

- Visual acuity test. This eye chart test measures how well you see at various distances.
- Dilated eye exam. Drops are placed in your eyes to widen, or dilate, the pupils. Your eye care professional uses a special magnifying lens to examine your retina and optic nerve for signs of damage and other eye problems. After the exam, your close-up vision may remain blurred for several hours.
- Tonometry. An instrument measures the pressure inside the eye. Numbing drops may be applied to your eye for this test.

Your eye care professional checks your retina for early signs of the disease, including:

- Leaking blood vessels.
- Retinal swelling (macular edema).
- Pale, fatty deposits on the retina—signs of leaking blood vessels.
- Damaged nerve tissue.
- Any changes to the blood vessels.

If your eye care professional believes you need treatment for macular edema, he or she may suggest a *fluorescein angiogram*. In this test, a special dye is injected into your arm. Pictures are taken as the dye passes through the blood vessels in your retina. The test allows your eye care professional to identify any leaking blood vessels and recommend treatment.

How Is Macular Edema Treated?

Macular edema is treated with laser surgery. This procedure is called focal laser treatment. Your doctor places up to several hundred small laser burns in the areas of retinal leakage surrounding the macula. These burns slow the leakage of fluid and reduce the amount of fluid in the retina. The surgery is usually completed in one session. Further treatment may be needed.

A patient may need focal laser surgery more than once to control the leaking fluid. If you have macular edema in both eyes and require laser surgery, generally only one eye will be treated at a time, usually several weeks apart.

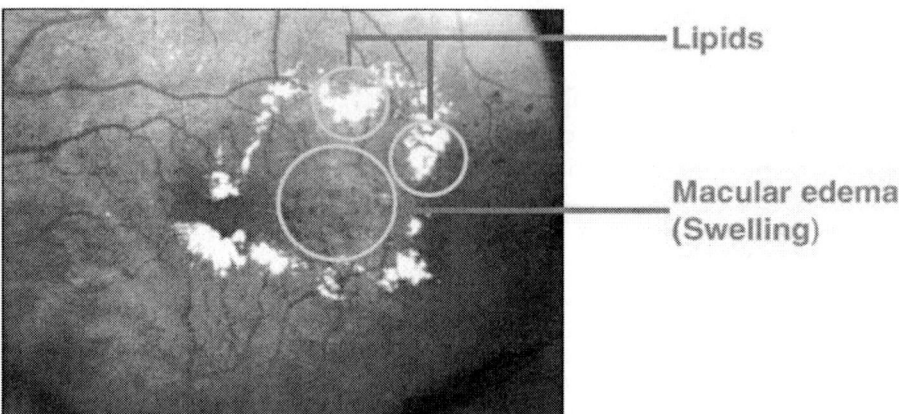
The retina prior to focal laser treatment

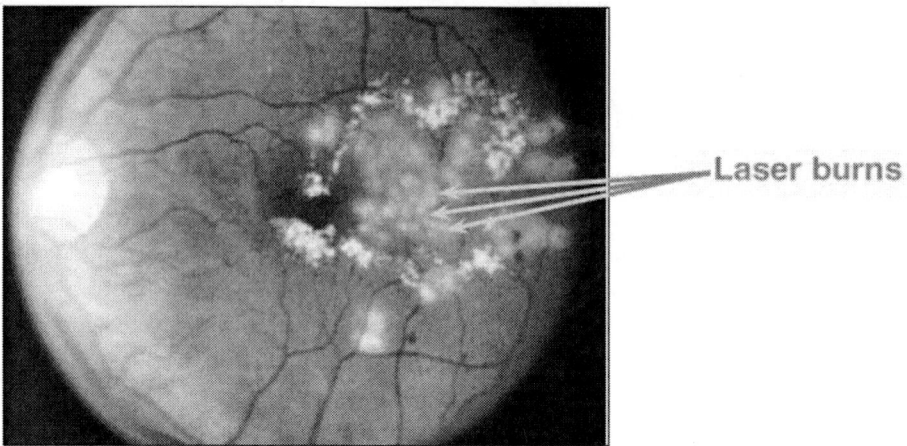
The retina immediately after focal laser treatment

Focal laser treatment stabilizes vision. In fact, focal laser treatment reduces the risk of vision loss by 50 percent. In a small number of cases, if vision is lost, it can be improved. Contact your eye care professional if you have vision loss.

How Is Diabetic Retinopathy Treated?

During the first three stages of diabetic retinopathy, no treatment is needed, unless you have macular edema. To prevent progression of diabetic retinopathy, people with diabetes should control their levels of blood sugar, blood pressure, and blood cholesterol.

Proliferative retinopathy is treated with laser surgery. This procedure is called scatter laser treatment. Scatter laser treatment helps to shrink the abnormal blood vessels. Your doctor places 1,000 to 2,000 laser burns in the areas of the retina away from the macula, causing the abnormal blood vessels to shrink. Because a high number of laser burns are necessary, two or more sessions usually are required to complete treatment. Although you may notice some loss of your side vision, scatter laser treatment can save the rest of your sight. Scatter laser treatment may slightly reduce your color vision and night vision.

Scatter laser treatment works better before the fragile, new blood vessels have started to bleed. That is why it is important to have regular, comprehensive dilated eye exams. Even if bleeding has started, scatter laser treatment may still be possible, depending on the amount of bleeding.

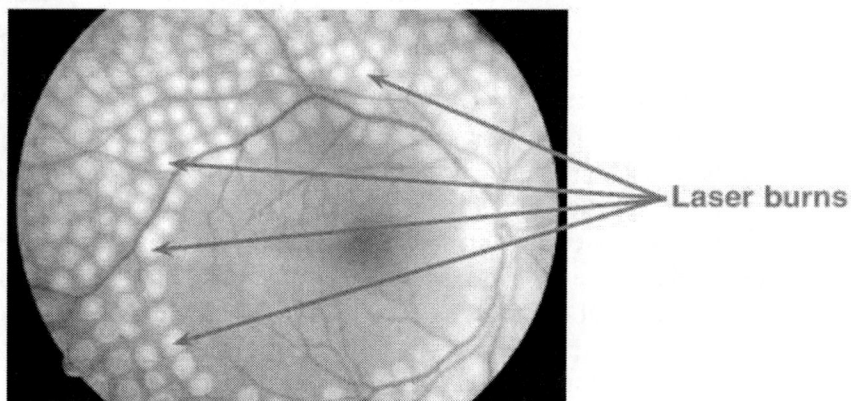

Scatter laser treatment

If the bleeding is severe, you may need a surgical procedure called a vitrectomy (described on the next page). During a vitrectomy, blood is removed from the center of your eye.

What Happens during Laser Treatment?

Both focal and scatter laser treatment are performed in your doctor's office or eye clinic. Before the surgery, your doctor will dilate your pupil and apply drops to numb the eye. The area behind your eye also may be numbed to prevent discomfort.

The lights in the office will be dim. As you sit facing the laser machine, your doctor will hold a special lens to your eye. During the procedure, you may see flashes of light. These flashes eventually may create a stinging sensation that can be uncomfortable.

You will need someone to drive you home after surgery. Because your pupil will remain dilated for a few hours, you should bring a pair of sunglasses.

For the rest of the day, your vision will probably be a little blurry. If your eye hurts, your doctor can suggest treatment.

What Is a Vitrectomy?

If you have a lot of blood in the center of the eye (vitreous gel), you may need a vitrectomy to restore your sight. If you need vitrectomies in both eyes, they are usually done several weeks apart.

A vitrectomy is performed under either local or general anesthesia. Your doctor makes a tiny incision in your eye. Next, a small instrument is used to remove the vitreous gel that is clouded with blood. The vitreous gel is replaced with a salt solution. Because the vitreous gel is mostly water, you will notice no change between the salt solution and the original vitreous gel.

You will probably be able to return home after the vitrectomy. Some people stay in the hospital overnight. Your eye will be red and sensitive. You will need to wear an eye patch for a few days or weeks to protect your eye. You also will need to use medicated eyedrops to protect against infection.

Are Scatter Laser Treatment and Vitrectomy Effective in Treating Proliferative Retinopathy?

Yes. Both treatments are very effective in reducing vision loss. People with proliferative retinopathy have less than a five percent chance of becoming blind within five years when they get timely and appropriate treatment. Although both treatments have high success rates, they do not cure diabetic retinopathy.

Once you have proliferative retinopathy, you always will be at risk for new bleeding. You may need treatment more than once to protect your sight.

What Can I Do if I Already Have Lost Some Vision from Diabetic Retinopathy?

If you have lost some sight from diabetic retinopathy, ask your eye care professional about low vision services and devices that may help you make the most of your remaining vision. Ask for a referral to a specialist in low vision. Many community organizations and agencies offer information about low vision counseling, training, and other special services for people with visual impairments. A nearby school of medicine or optometry may provide low vision services.

What Research Is Being Done?

The National Eye Institute (NEI) is conducting and supporting research that seeks better ways to detect, treat, and prevent vision loss in people with diabetes. This research is conducted through studies in the laboratory and with patients.

For example, researchers are studying drugs that may stop the retina from sending signals to the body to grow new blood vessels. Someday, these drugs may help people control their diabetic retinopathy and reduce the need for laser surgery.

What Can I Do to Protect My Vision?

The NEI urges everyone with diabetes to have a comprehensive dilated eye exam at least once a year. If you have diabetic retinopathy, you may need an eye exam more often. People with proliferative retinopathy can reduce their risk of blindness by 95 percent with timely treatment and appropriate followup care.

A major study has shown that better control of blood sugar levels slows the onset and progression of retinopathy. The people with diabetes who kept their blood sugar levels as close to normal as possible also had much less kidney and nerve disease. Better control also reduces the need for sight-saving laser surgery.

This level of blood sugar control may not be best for everyone, including some elderly patients, children under age 13, or people with heart disease. Be sure to ask your doctor if such a control program is right for you.

Other studies have shown that controlling elevated blood pressure and cholesterol can reduce the risk of vision loss. Controlling these will help your overall health as well as help protect your vision.

What Should I Ask My Eye Care Professional?

You can protect yourself against vision loss by working in partnership with your eye care professional. Ask questions and get the information you need to take care of yourself and your family.

What Are Some Questions to Ask?

About My Eye Disease or Disorder...

- What is my diagnosis?
- What caused my condition?
- Can my condition be treated?
- How will this condition affect my vision now and in the future?
- Should I watch for any particular symptoms and notify you if they occur?
- Should I make any lifestyle changes?

About My Treatment...

- What is the treatment for my condition?
- When will the treatment start and how long will it last?
- What are the benefits of this treatment and how successful is it?
- What are the risks and side effects associated with this treatment?

- Are there foods, drugs, or activities I should avoid while I'm on this treatment?
- If my treatment includes taking medicine, what should I do if I miss a dose?
- Are other treatments available?

About My Tests...

- What kinds of tests will I have?
- What can I expect to find out from these tests?
- When will I know the results?
- Do I have to do anything special to prepare for any of the tests?
- Do these tests have any side effects or risks?
- Will I need more tests later?

Other Suggestions

- If you don't understand your eye care professional's responses, ask questions until you do understand.
- Take notes or get a friend or family member to take notes for you. Or, bring a tape recorder to help you remember the discussion.
- Ask your eye care professional to write down his or her instructions to you.
- Ask your eye care professional for printed material about your condition.
- If you still have trouble understanding your eye care professional's answers, ask where you can go for more information.
- Other members of your health care team, such as nurses and pharmacists, can be good sources of information. Talk to them, too.

Today, patients take an active role in their health care. Be an active patient about your eye care.

Remember ...

If you have diabetes, get a comprehensive dilated eye exam *at least once a year.*

- Proliferative retinopathy can develop without symptoms. At this advanced stage, you are at high risk for vision loss.
- Macular edema can develop without symptoms at any of the four stages of diabetic retinopathy.
- You can develop both proliferative retinopathy and macular edema and still see fine. However, you are at high risk for vision loss.

Your eye care professional can tell if you have macular edema or any stage of diabetic retinopathy. Whether or not you have symptoms, early detection and timely treatment can prevent vision loss.

Where Can I Get More Information?

For more information about diabetic retinopathy or diabetes, you may wish to contact:

American Academy of Ophthalmology*
P.O. Box 7424
San Francisco, CA 94120–7424
415–561–8500
www.aao.org

American Optometric Association*
243 North Lindbergh Boulevard
St. Louis, MO 63141–7851
314–991–4100
www.aoa.org

American Diabetes Association
1701 North Beauregard Street Alexandria,
VA 22311–1717 1–800–342–2383 (National Headquarters)
1–888–342–2383 (Local Offices) 703–549–1500
E-mail: AskADA@diabetes.org

www.diabetes.org
Juvenile Diabetes Research Foundation International
120 Wall Street
New York, NY 10005–4001
1–800–533–CURE (2873)
E-mail: info@jdrf.org
www.jdrf.org

National Diabetes Information Clearinghouse
1 Information Way
Bethesda, MD 20892–3560
1–800–860–8747
301–654–3327
E-mail: ndic@info.niddk.nih.gov
www.niddk.nih.gov

National Eye Institute*
National Institutes of Health 2020 Vision Place
Bethesda, MD 20892–3655
301–496–5248
E-mail: 2020@nei.nih.gov
www.nei.nih.gov

Prevent Blindness America*
211 West Wacker Drive, 17th Floor Chicago, IL 60606
1-800-331-2020; ext. 6026
312-363-6026
E-mail: info@preventblindness.org
www.preventblindness.org

* These organizations also provide information on low vision.

For more information about low vision programs, you may wish to contact:
American Foundation for the Blind
11 Penn Plaza, Suite 300
New York, NY 10001–2006
1–800–232–5463; 212–502–7600
E-mail: afbinfo@afb.net

www.afb.org
Council of Citizens with Low Vision International
1–800–733–2258
Lighthouse International 111 East 59th Street
New York, NY 10022–1202
1–800–334–5497
1–800–829–0500
212–821–9200
212–821–9713 (TDD)
E-mail: info@lighthouse.org
www.lighthouse.org

National Association for Visually Handicapped
22 West 21st Street, 6th Floor
New York, NY 10010–6493
212–889–3141
www.navh.org

Index

A

African Americans, 4, 11, 12, 33
age, vii, 4, 11, 12, 17, 18, 19, 22, 23, 26, 31, 32, 33, 36, 44, 56
agencies, 13, 55
age-related cataract, vii, 19, 26
age-related macular degeneration, vii, 22, 23, 26, 31, 44
alcohol use, 20
allergic reaction, 35
AMD, vii, 31, 32, 33, 34, 35, 36, 37, 38, 39, 40, 42, 43, 44
anatomy, 4
angiogram, 35, 51
antibiotic, 39
anxiety, 32
atrophy, 36

B

benefits, 12, 22, 23, 27, 40, 56
beta-carotene, 37, 38
bleeding, 23, 24, 25, 50, 53, 55
blind spot, 40
blindness, 1, 16, 32, 45, 47, 48, 50, 55
blood pressure, 3, 10, 33, 53, 56
blood supply, 48
blood vessels, 35, 36, 39, 47, 48, 49, 51, 53, 55
brain, 2, 18, 33, 36, 42

C

caregivers, 43
carotene, 38
cataract(s), vii, 9, 10, 11, 17, 18, 19, 20, 21, 22, 23, 24, 25, 26, 28
Caucasians, 33
Chicago, 14, 29, 46, 59
childhood, 21
children, 10, 56
cholesterol, 33, 53, 56
closure, 10
coherence, 35
color, 25, 35, 53
common symptoms, 20
community, 13, 43, 55
complications, 11, 35
cooking, 32, 40, 42
copper, 37, 38
cornea, 2, 4, 6, 10, 23
cost, 39
counseling, 13, 55
cure, 6, 38, 39, 54

D

daily living, 41
damages, 11, 47
Department of Health and Human Services, 16
deposits, 35, 51
depression, 43
detachment, 23
detection, 1, 37, 58
diabetes, 11, 12, 18, 20, 21, 47, 49, 53, 55, 58
diabetic retinopathy, vii, 22, 47, 49, 50, 52, 54, 55, 58
diet, 33
discomfort, 24, 54
diseases, 1, 11, 20, 26
disorder, vii, 27
drainage, 2, 8, 9, 10, 11
drugs, 11, 27, 39, 40, 55, 57
drusen, 35, 36

E

early warning, 49
edema, 49, 50, 51, 52, 58
emergency, 10, 23
environment, 20
exercise, 37
exposure, 20, 21, 26
eye disease, vii, 26, 27

F

families, vii, 1
family history, 4, 11, 12, 33, 36
family members, 11, 43
fatty acids, 37, 38
filtration, 8
fish, 33, 37, 38
fish oil, 38
floaters, 23
fluid, 2, 7, 8, 10, 11, 24, 36, 49, 51
Food and Drug Administration (FDA), 29

G

gel, 48, 54
general anesthesia, 54
genes, 11
glasses, 25, 40, 41
glaucoma, vii, 1, 2, 3, 4, 5, 6, 7, 8, 10, 11, 12, 13, 14, 15, 21, 23, 26
glaucoma surgery, 11
growth, 39, 48
guidance, 41

H

hallucinations, 42
healing, 24, 25
health care, 13, 28, 57
health problems, 21
heart disease, 56
high blood pressure, 11
Hispanics, 4, 33

I

image(s), 17, 18, 19, 20, 33, 35, 42
impairments, 13, 55
independence, 41
infants, 10
infection, 9, 10, 23, 24, 25, 39, 54
inflammation, 8, 9, 10, 25
ingredients, 38
injections, 8, 39
injury(s), 11, 21
iris, 2, 10, 11, 18, 35
isolation, 43

K

kidney, 56

L

landscapes, 42
Latinos, 4, 33
lead, 32, 36, 43
leakage, 51
learning, 43
learning skills, 43
lens, 6, 8, 17, 18, 19, 21, 22, 25, 34, 51, 54
lifestyle changes, 12, 27, 36, 56
light, 2, 8, 10, 17, 18, 19, 24, 25, 33, 35, 36, 42, 47, 54
light beam, 35
lung cancer, 38
lutein, 37, 38

M

macular degeneration, vii, 22, 23, 26, 31, 44
materials, 41
measurement, 6
medical, 3, 10, 11, 23, 24, 25, 43
medical history, 10
Medicare, 12, 41
medication, 15
medicine, 7, 8, 11, 12, 15, 27, 40, 55, 57
mental illness, 42
milligrams, 38
myopia, 23

N

National Institutes of Health, 1, 14, 16, 17, 28, 31, 45, 47, 59
nausea, 10, 35
nearsightedness, 23
nerve, 2, 18, 51, 56
nerve fibers, 2
nurses, 13, 28, 57
nutrients, 38
nutrition, 26

O

occupational therapy, 41
omega-3, 37, 38
open-angle glaucoma, vii, 1, 2, 3, 4, 6, 10
operations, 9, 22
ophthalmologist, 35, 40
optic nerve, 1, 2, 3, 4, 6, 10, 21, 33, 34, 51
outpatient, 25

P

pain, 4, 10, 23, 25
pregnancy, 49
prevention, 37

R

radiation, 21
reactions, 43
reading, 22, 41, 42
rehabilitation program, 41
researchers, 11, 55
resources, 41, 42, 43
retina, 2, 6, 17, 18, 19, 21, 23, 32, 33, 34, 35, 36, 39, 40, 47, 48, 51, 52, 53, 55
retinal detachment, 23
retinopathy, vii, 47, 48, 49, 50, 53, 54, 55, 58
risk(s), 2, 3, 4, 10, 11, 12, 13, 15, 16, 20, 22, 23, 24, 26, 27, 33, 36, 37, 38, 39, 40, 49, 52, 55, 56, 57, 58
risk factors, 4, 10, 20, 33

S

scatter, 53
self-esteem, 43
sensation, 54
sensing, 33
sensitivity, 10
services, 13, 15, 31, 40, 41, 55
shade, 19

shape, 23
side effects, 7, 8, 10, 12, 13, 15, 16, 27, 40, 56, 57
signals, 18, 33, 48, 55
signs, 6, 21, 26, 34, 37, 49, 51
smoking, 20, 33, 37, 38
social workers, 41
success rate, 54
swelling, 25, 36, 48, 51
symptoms, vii, 1, 4, 8, 10, 12, 20, 22, 27, 31, 33, 36, 37, 48, 49, 56, 58
syndrome, 42

T

TDD, 15, 45, 60
tension, 3, 10
therapy, 39, 41
tissue, 2, 8, 17, 25, 36, 39, 47, 51
training, 13, 41, 42, 55
treatment, vii, 1, 5, 6, 7, 8, 10, 11, 12, 22, 23, 24, 26, 27, 35, 37, 39, 40, 43, 49, 50, 51, 52, 53, 54, 55, 56, 57, 58
trial, 37, 38
tumors, 11

U

ultrasound, 35
United States, 22
uveitis, 11

V

vascular endothelial growth factor (VEGF), 39
vegetables, 26, 33, 37, 38
vein, 39
vessels, 35, 36, 39, 48, 49, 51, 53
vision, 1, 2, 4, 5, 6, 7, 10, 11, 12, 13, 15, 17, 19, 20, 21, 22, 23, 25, 26, 27, 29, 31, 32, 33, 34, 35, 36, 37, 38, 39, 40, 41, 42, 43, 46, 47, 48, 49, 50, 51, 52, 53, 54, 55, 56, 58, 59
visual images, 42
vitamin C, 37, 38
vitamin E, 37, 38
vitamins, 37, 38

W

watches, 41
water, 18, 19, 54
wear, 8, 18, 24, 54

Z

zinc, 37, 38
zinc oxide, 38